Amel Ben Hamad
Nadia Kolsi
Rania Gargouri

HYPETROPHIC CARDIOMYOPATHY IN NEWBORNS AND MATERNAL DIABETES

Amel Ben Hamad
Nadia Kolsi
Rania Gargouri

HYPETROPHIC CARDIOMYOPATHY IN NEWBORNS AND MATERNAL DIABETES

ScienciaScripts

Imprint

Cover image: www.ingimage.com

This book is a translation from the original published under ISBN 978-620-6-72199-4.

Publisher:
Sciencia Scripts
is a trademark of
Dodo Books Indian Ocean Ltd. and OmniScriptum S.R.L publishing group

120 High Road, East Finchley, London, N2 9ED, United Kingdom
Str. Armeneasca 28/1, office 1, Chisinau MD-2012, Republic of Moldova, Europe
Printed at: see last page
ISBN: 978-620-8-09030-2

PLAN

INTRODUCTION

Newborns born to diabetic mothers (NNMD) represent a high-risk group of newborns, with an increased incidence of perinatal morbidity and mortality. The mortality rate is estimated at 13.9/1000 live births, compared with 7/1000 live births for babies born to non-diabetic mothers. NNMD also have a higher rate of admission to intensive care (10% compared with 3%) (1).

These newborns run an increased risk of macrosomia, hypoglycaemia, hypocalcaemia, cardiovascular abnormalities and respiratory distress syndrome.

Approximately 3-6% of NNMD suffer from cardiovascular abnormalities. Hypertrophic cardiomyopathy (HCM) is the most common cardiac disorder, accounting for 40% of cardiovascular anomalies (2). Its incidence, often underestimated due to the frequency of asymptomatic forms, varies between 30% and 40% (3).

NNMD HCM is characterised by disproportionate hypertrophy of the heart: hypertrophy of the interventricular septum (IVS) and free ventricular walls. Histology of the myocardium shows hypertrophy of muscle fibres with increased mass of myocardial nuclei and sarcoplasm (4).

This particular form of MHC is mainly induced by foetal hyperinsulinism secondary to maternal hyperglycaemia. It manifests as cardiac hypertrophy, preferentially affecting the SIV due to its high insulin receptor content (5).

The manifestations of HCM can vary considerably, ranging from a simple echocardiographic finding of no particular clinical significance, to congestive heart failure due to obstruction of the left ventricular ejection pathway. Whatever its severity, cardiac hypertrophy is transient, with echocardiographic resolution around six months of age in all cases (6).

Several studies have suggested that maintaining strict control of maternal glycaemia can reduce the incidence of cardiovascular anomalies. A beneficial effect on the incidence of congenital heart defects has been observed. However, it appears that strict control of blood glucose levels has no significant effect on the development of HCM. This suggests that close cardiac monitoring of the fetus during pregnancies complicated by maternal diabetes may be essential to prevent serious perinatal complications (7).

IMPACT

1. Incidence

HCM is the most common cardiac condition in NNMD. Its incidence remains uncertain, as it is asymptomatic in most cases, and cardiac ultrasound is generally only performed if there is a clinical sign (17). According to most authors, HCM of NNMD affects 75% of foetuses in utero and 10 to 71% of newborns, with an estimated mean incidence of 30% (18,19) (Table LIX). Vela-huerta et al (20) compared term NNMD with term newborns of non-diabetic mothers in Mexico between July 2015 and March 2016. Two-dimensional echocardiography was performed within 24 hours of birth. Asymmetric septal hypertrophy was present only in NNMDs (50% versus 0%). SIV thickness and the SIV/PPVG thickness ratio were also significantly higher in the first group.Vela and Huerta et al (1) also carried out a study between January and December 1997. 80 NNMD (group A) and 85 macrosomic newborns of non-diabetic mothers (group B) were included. As a control group (group C), 85 healthy eutrophic newborns born at term were studied. HCM was present in 33 newborns (38.8%) in group A, in 6 newborns (7.1%) in group B and in no newborns in group C. These differences were statistically significant.

Table I: Incidence of hypertrophic cardiomyopathy in newborns of diabetic mothers according to series in the literature

series	Years	Country	Number of cases	Case of hypertrophic cardiomyopathy
Bogo et al. (21)	2018	Brazil	48	3 (6%)
Vela-huerta2015- Mexico et al (20)2016			38	19 (50%)
By 2009- HăşmăşanuRomania 2012 et al (22)			35	10 (28,57%)
Russell and2008 Ireland al.(3)			26	5 (22%)
El- 2007- GanzouryEgypt 2008			69	30 (43,5%)
et al (23)				
Ben Hamida	2006	Tunisia	33	18 (54%)
Hayet (11)				
Abu- 2000-Arabia- Sulaiman and 2001Saudi al.(24)			100	38 (38%)
Vela Huerta 1997Mexico et al (1)			80	33 (38,8%)
Jeaggi et al.1994-Canada (25)1996			45	15 (33%)

CHARACTERISTICS

2. Features

2.1.Age maternal

Pregnant women with type 2 diabetes or GDM tend to be older. In Australia, among women with diabetes who gave birth between 2005 and 2008, the maternal age pattern was 30-34 years. Women who gave birth with GDM and those with PPG were more likely to be older (30 years and over) than women who gave birth without diabetes (70%, 65% and 54% respectively). Around 71% of mothers with type 2 diabetes or GDM were aged 30 years and over compared with around 55% of mothers with type 1 diabetes or no diabetes during pregnancy (26).

2.2.Parity

In Australia, women with gestational diabetes (59%) were more likely to be multiparous than those with gestational diabetes (56%). Mothers with gestational diabetes were less likely to be multiparous than those without diabetes (58%) (26).

2.3.Weight maternal

In line with trends in the general population, the rate and severity of maternal obesity has increased in recent years (27). In European countries, between 7% and 25% of mothers-to-be are overweight (28). In the United States, only 45% of mothers are of normal weight when they become pregnant (29).

Maternal obesity is a risk factor for the development of GDM and type 2 diabetes (27).

2.4. Morbidity maternal

2.4.1. Diabetes maternal

Maternal diabetes can be pre-gestational, diagnosed before pregnancy (type 1 or type 2 diabetes), or gestational, diagnosed during pregnancy (30). It is a condition frequently found during pregnancy, with an estimated incidence of 7%. Insulin-dependent GDM affects 0.5 to 2% of pregnancies, whereas GDM affects approximately 1.2 to 7.2% (18,31). According to the 2016 World Health Organisation report on diabetes, the prevalence of diabetes has doubled over the last four decades, with a decrease in the age of onset of the disease (32). As a result, pregnancies complicated by maternal diabetes are expected to occur more frequently.The International Diabetes Federation estimated that 20.9 million, or 16.2%, of newborns born in 2015 were exposed to some form of maternal hyperglycaemia during pregnancy. 85.1% of these were from pregnancies complicated by GDM, 7.4% from other types of diabetes detected for the first time during pregnancy and 7.5% from maternal diabetes detected before pregnancy, known as DPG (10).In Norway, between 1994 and 2009, 5618 (0.61%) of the 914427 registered births (live births, stillbirths, interrupted pregnancies) were complicated by gestational diabetes and 9726 (1.06%) by gestational diabetes (33). In Australia, between 2005 and 2007, more than 5% of pregnancies were complicated by diabetes. Less than 1% of mothers had gestational diabetes and around 5% had gestational diabetes (26).In the United States, diabetes mellitus currently complicates around 10% of all pregnancies (34). In a large study conducted in California, the incidence of GDM rose from 1.3% in 1999 to 1.82% in 2005 (35). In In the same cohort, FGD affected 7.5% of pregnancies in 1999 and 7.4% in 2005.

➢ **Pre-gestational diabetes**

The incidence of GDM is increasing due to the epidemic of childhood obesity. When obese children reach childbearing age, more and more women are diagnosed with type 2 diabetes before pregnancy (3,31).

➢ **Gestational diabetes**

GDM has been defined as any degree of glucose intolerance that first appears or is recognised during pregnancy. Therefore, the diagnosis of GDM includes both an abnormality of glucose intolerance undiagnosed before pregnancy and pregnancy-related glucose intolerance that disappears after delivery. However, a definitive diagnosis can only be made in the post-partum period (8).

The prevalence of GDM has increased worldwide. The incidence is estimated at between 2 and 6%. It varies from country to country, and may reach 20% in certain populations (36,37). It has been reported to range from 3 to 14% worldwide, and from 3 to 5% in North America, Europe and Australia (26). In France, it is estimated at between 6 and 7% according to the 2010 perinatal survey (38).A recent meta-analysis in India showed that the average prevalence of GDM is 10.1%, with an upward trend from 0.53% to 27.3% (39,40).

3. Pregnancy And Childbirth

3.1.Pregnancy follow-up

3.1.1. Obstetrical ultrasound antenatal

Pregnancy in diabetic women is often complicated by hydramnios. In our series, hydramnios was noted in 32% of mothers. In the literature, an association has been noted between blood flow in the ductus Arantius and cardiac function (41). Increased values of the pulsatility index and the absence or reversal of flow in the ductus Arantius during atrial contraction have been correlated with unfavourable pregnancy outcomes (42). Zielinsky et al (43) studied 56 fetuses of diabetic mothers, 20 of whom had HCM, and 53 healthy fetuses of non-diabetic mothers. Fetuses with septal hypertrophy had a significantly higher pulsatility index than those without hypertrophy and control fetuses from non-diabetic mothers.

3.1.2. Fetal cardiac ultrasound

3.1.2.1. Technical interest and

Fetal cardiac ultrasound is a non-invasive, accessible and accurate screening tool widely used to assess cardiac structure and function (44,45). Fetal cardiac ultrasound, including cross-sectioning of the four chambers of the heart, cross-sectioning of the ejection tract and cross-sectioning of the three vessels and trachea, is part of routine anatomical screening. But cardiac assessment in diabetic mothers must also include the visceral situs. atrial, foramen ovale, systemic and pulmonary venous connections, atrioventricular and ventriculoarterial connections, aortic arches and superior and inferior vena cava, with and without colour mapping (46). Conventionally, fetal heart ultrasound is usually performed for high-risk populations during morphological ultrasound between 18ème and 22ème weeks of amenorrhoea. However, with advances in ultrasound technology and growing experience of fetal heart ultrasound, the end of the first trimester has been recognised as a plausible time to perform this examination (46,47). The trans-abdominal and trans-vaginal routes are the most recommended methods (48).Fetal cardiomyopathies can be analysed by studying atrial and ventricular contraction using B and M mode echocardiography.

3.1.2.2. Anomalies detected

The in-utero manifestations of myocardial hypertrophy are not always striking. However, hypertrophy is easily detected by standard fetal echocardiography, usually by comparing SIV thickness with established nomograms: an increase in parietal thickness above 97.5% of normal values for gestational age (49,50).
SIV hypertrophy with values greater than 2 DS is predominant at all gestational ages (Figure 37). Cardiac function is impaired between 24 and 27 weeks' gestation (44). However, HCM may not appear until the last trimester of pregnancy, without necessarily altering myocardial function (21).

Diastolic dysfunction in fetuses of diabetic mothers coexists often with an increase in the thickness of the ventricular wall (51). However, it may precede myocardial hypertrophy (50) or be completely independent of it (52).

The myocardial performance index, between 27ème and 40ème weeks of amenorrhoea, in the foetuses of diabetic mothers is significantly higher than in those of non-diabetic mothers. This is probably due to impaired myocardial performance at the end of pregnancy and to changes in myocardial maturation and development (21,53,54).

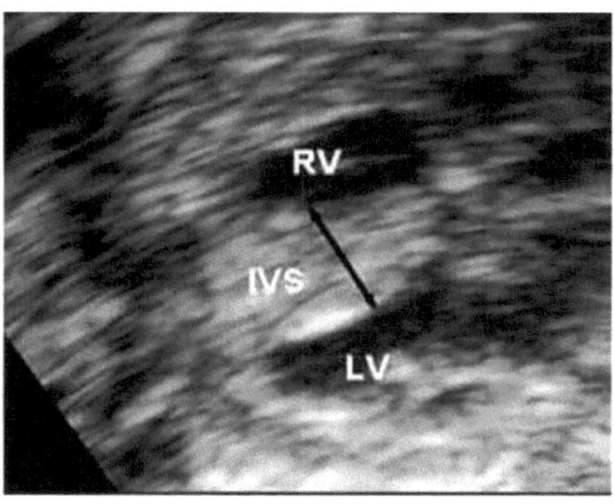

Figure 1: Severe septal hypertrophy in a 33-week-old foetus of a diabetic mother (black arrow = interventricular septum) (50)

3.1.2.3. Data from literature

In the study by Garg et al (44), 302 pregnant women with diabetes and 294 pregnant women without diabetes underwent foetal echocardiography. SIV and PPVG thicknesses were significantly higher in the foetuses of diabetic mothers. Diastolic function was impaired in the foetuses of women with GDM. Bogo et al (21) studied the thickness of the SIV prenatally and postnatally in 48 newborns from pregnancies complicated by GD. SIV hypertrophy was noted in 14 fetuses (29%). The shortening fraction was normal in 100% of cases. Rossi Palmieri et al (19) studied fetal cardiac ultrasound data in 63 pregnant women whose pregnancies were complicated by GD between July and December 2013. SIV thickness was greater than 2 DS in 50.8% of fetuses, between 1 and 2 in 38.09% of fetuses and less than 1 DS in 11.11% of fetuses. The thickness of the PPVG was greater than 2 DS in 13 fetuses (20.6%). HCM was confirmed in 54% of fetuses.Fouda et al (55) studied fetal echocardiography data in 119 pregnant women. They were divided into 3 groups: 32 non-diabetic, 47 followed for PPG and 40 who developed gestational diabetes. The SIV was significantly thicker in both groups of diabetic mothers compared with the control group. In addition, the SIV was significantly thicker in the PGD group compared with the GDM group. Ten fetuses in the DPG group and four fetuses in the DG group had a SIV thickness greater than 5 mm. Fourteen fetuses of diabetic mothers had septal hypertrophy (16.09%). There was no statistically significant difference between left and right ventricular wall thickness in the three groups. In a study by Zielinsky et al (56), 42 mothers with gestational diabetes and 39 mothers without diabetes underwent fetal echocardiography. The mean left atrial shortening was significantly lower in the fetuses of diabetic mothers than in those of the control group. They concluded that foetuses of mothers with previous GDM or GD have impaired left ventricular diastolic function.

3.2. Delivery route

NNMD are at greater risk of being born by caesarean section (57,58). In Australia, mothers with GDM were more likely to have a preterm birth, induced preterm labour and a caesarean section than mothers with GDM or no diabetes during pregnancy. Mothers with GDM were at greater risk of preterm induced labour and caesarean section than those without diabetes during pregnancy (26). El-Ganzoury et al (23) studied 69 NNMD. 57 were born by caesarean section (82.6%) and 12 by vaginal delivery (17.4%). Yang et al (59) compared foetal and neonatal outcomes between 516 NNMD and 150,589 neonates born to non-diabetic mothers. The caesarean delivery rate in the general population was high, but it was particularly high in NNMD (49.0% versus 19.5%). Macrosomic

NNMD were no more likely to give birth by caesarean section than non-macrosomic NNMD. Diabetic women who gave birth vaginally were more likely than non-diabetic women to require forceps or vacuum assistance.

4. Characteristics of newborns

4.1.Gender

We did not find any data in the literature concerning gender predominance in NNMD MHC.

4.2.Term of delivery

Diabetes during pregnancy is associated with a risk of premature birth estimated to be two to three times higher than in non-diabetic women (60). In a series by Cordero et al (61) including 322 newborns of women with GDM and 177 newborns of women with insulin-dependent GDM, 36% were born prematurely (14% before 34ème weeks of amenorrhoea and 22% between 34ème and 37ème weeks of amenorrhoea). In the study by Ullmo et al (7) of 87 pregnancies complicated by maternal diabetes, preterm delivery was noted in 34 of the 87 pregnancies, two of which were due to severe HCM.

4.3.Adaptation to life outside the uterus

FHR abnormalities and perinatal asphyxia may occur in 25% of NNMD. They are related to atherosclerosis in the mother, hyperglycaemia (before delivery but especially during labour), and the frequently observed premature delivery (62).
In Australia, newborns of mothers with CPB have higher rates of stillbirth, preterm birth, high birth weight, low Apgar score, heavy resuscitation, admission to a special care nursery or neonatal intensive care unit than newborns of mothers with GDM or without diabetes during pregnancy (26).

4.4. Birth weight

4.4.1. Incidence of macrosomia in newborns of diabetic mothers

NNMDs have anthropometric indices of weight, height and head circumference above the 90ème percentile (57). Excess adiposity in NNMD is essentially due to maternal hyperglycaemia, which produces foetal hyperglycaemia followed by increased insulin secretion by the foetus. This anabolic hormone increases the synthesis of proteins, lipids and carbohydrates. In the presence of increased substrates, foetal hyperinsulinaemia causes macrosomia and organomegaly (57). In the study by Yang et al (59), the rate of macrosomic NNMD was high, at 45.2%, compared with 12.6% in newborns of non-diabetic mothers. 24 of the 92 NNMD were macrosomic in the study by Ullmo et al (7). Persson et al (63) reported an incidence of 31% of macrosomic newborns in a cohort of over 5000 newborns born to mothers with type 1 diabetes in Sweden between 1991 and 2003.In another study, Persson et al (64) reported an incidence of macrosomia of 47% in 3705 newborns born to mothers with type 1 diabetes in Sweden between 1998 and 2007. Birth weight was greater than 4500 g in 14% of the population. In the study conducted by Hăşmăşanu et al (22), 35 NNMD (DPG and DG) and 35 control neonates, born between January 2009 and December 2012 in Cluj-Napoca (north-west Romania), were collated. The mean weight of the NNMDs (3695.57 gr ± 738.63 gr) was significantly higher than the mean weight of the newborns of non-diabetic mothers (3276.14 gr ± 496.51 gr).

4.4.2. Factors associated with macrosomia

4.4.2.1. Type of diabetes maternal

Maternal diabetes has been shown to be associated with neonatal macrosomia. Diabetic mothers go through intermittent periods of hyperglycaemia resulting in foetal hyperglycaemia which stimulates the production of growth factors. These factors stimulate foetal growth by depositing glycogen and fat, leading to macrosomia (23). According to a large study carried out in the United Kingdom

(58), women with gestational diabetes were twice as likely to have a baby weighing more than 4000g at birth compared with the general population (21% compared with 11%). There was no difference in birth weight between babies born to women with type 1 or type 2 diabetes mellitus (57,58). Newborns of mothers with GDM are 2.5 times more likely to be macrosomic compared with the general population (65). Lindsay et al (66) found that babies born to mothers with GDM had significantly higher birth weights. Åman et al (67) studied the birth weight of 56 newborns: 18 from mothers with well-controlled type 1 diabetes, 10 from mothers who had developed GDM, and 28 control newborns. The mean birth weight of newborns from mothers with type 1 diabetes was equal to that of newborns from mothers with GDM, although birth weight appeared to be higher in the type 1 diabetes group due to a shorter gestational age. The prevalence rate of birth weight adjusted for gestational age and sex above the 90ème percentile was 56, 30 and 11% in newborns of mothers with type 1 diabetes, mothers with GDM and control newborns, respectively.

4.4.2.2. Diabetes control maternal

The rate of foetal macrosomia remains high despite good control of diabetes (64). The risk of macrosomia increases when the mother's mean glucose concentration chronically exceeds 1.30g/l. This risk is even higher when the mother's glucose concentrations are episodically high, particularly after a meal (pulsatile hyperglycaemia) (62). In the study conducted by Åman et al (67), no association was found between maternal HbA1c at the beginning (6 to 12 weeks of amenorrhoea) or at the end of pregnancy (24, 28, 32 or 36 weeks of amenorrhoea) and birth weight (67). El-Ganzoury et al (23) studied the birth weight of 69 NNMD. 22 newborns were born to mothers with optimal diabetes control (HbA1c less than 7%), all of whom were eutrophic. 47 were born to mothers with poorly controlled diabetes (maternal HbA1c greater than or equal to 7%); these included all hypotrophic and macrosomic neonates and three eutrophic neonates.

4.4.2.3. Weight maternal

Maternal obesity is a recognised risk factor for fetal macrosomia (68,69). In our series, we found a positive correlation between maternal weight at the end of pregnancy and the trophicity of the newborn ($p = 0.018$). In the study conducted by Åman et al (67), no association was observed between birth weight and maternal weight.

CLINICAL PICTURE

5. Clinical

5.1. Signs physical

NNMD HCM is generally clinically silent, but 5-10% of newborns may be symptomatic (30). Severity may vary from incidental finding on echocardiography (30% of cases) to congestive heart failure (70,71). When the obstruction is severe, the newborn may present with respiratory distress, tachycardia, an ejection murmur and other signs of heart failure (1,63). This is due to systolic and diastolic myocardial dysfunction (51,72). Heart failure in the immediate postnatal period presents with tachypnoea, tachycardia, gallop rhythm and hepatomegaly. However, this is uncommon (12% of cases) and transient (70,71).Our results were comparable to those reported in the literature. Heart failure was found in only 4 newborns, i.e. 8% of cases. In the study by Ullmo et al (7), 12 of the 92 NNMD had HCF. Two deaths were noted. 9 newborns were symptomatic. Respiratory distress was present in 6 of them. Two had a murmur on cardiac auscultation. Cyanosis was noted in 2 newborns. In the study by Vela-Huerta et al (1), 7 of 33 NNMDs (21%) with HCM presented with signs of respiratory distress and a heart murmur. The symptoms resolved within the first 7 days of life, while the echocardiographic abnormalities disappeared within 2 months.

FURTHER TESTS

6. Additional examinations

6.1.Electrocardiogram

The ECG in NNMD may show sinus tachycardia, a prolonged corrected QT interval, changes in heart rate variability, a significant leftward shift of the electrical axis of the heart, ST segment and T wave changes and evidence of left or bi-ventricular hypertrophy (73,74).

The QT interval is an important electrophysiological marker that indicates the tendency towards ventricular arrhythmia and sudden cardiac death. A prolonged QT interval indicates regional differences in myocardial repolarisation. This may be associated with an increased risk of malignant ventricular tachyarrhythmias and sudden death, particularly in neonates with HCM (75).

These initial ECG abnormalities observed in NNMD generally disappear by six weeks of age. This period coincides with improvement in left ventricular hypertrophy and correction of metabolic disorders (75,76).

In the study by Vela-Huerta et al (1), ECG findings in NNMD with HCM were as follows: bi-ventricular hypertrophy in 55% of cases and right ventricular hypertrophy in 15% of cases.

Arslan et al (76) selected 47 newborns of mothers with GDM and 30 newborns of healthy mothers. The NNMD were classified according to SIV thickness: group 1 (16 newborns with septal hypertrophy), group 2 (31 newborns without septal hypertrophy) and group 3 (control group). The corrected QT was longer in group 1 than in groups 2 and 3. A highly significant positive correlation was detected between SIV end-diastolic thickness and corrected QT prolongation.

6.2.Chest X-ray

Cardiomegaly is common in NNMD. It is often associated with thickening of the IVS and subaortic stenosis in response to increased afterload (49). In the study by Vela-Huerta et al (1), the cardiothoracic index was 0.60 ± 0.1 in NNMD with HCM.Noirin et al (18) compared the heart weights of stillborn babies born to diabetic and non-diabetic mothers. They showed that those born to diabetic mothers had heavier hearts with thicker left ventricular walls without any disorganisation of the myocardial fibres. Jorgensen et al (77) studied cardiomegaly in 2083 stillborn babies. The most common association with cardiomegaly was maternal diabetes. The cohort included 68 NNMD, 39 of whom had a recorded cardiac weight. Cardiomegaly was found in 76.9% of all NNMD: 93% of those over 32 weeks' amenorrhoea and 100% of those over 40 weeks. However, it should be noted that cardiomegaly may be present in NNMD without HCM, due to persistent foetal circulation or a transient increase in arterial pressures. Neonatal hypoglycaemia, which is more common in NNMD, can lead to cardiomegaly and electrocardiographic abnormalities (70).

6.3.Cardiac ultrasound

HCM in NNMD is generally characterised by significant thickening of the SIV leading to reduced ventricular volumes and subsequent transient hypertrophic subaortic valve stenosis (7,30). Hypertrophy of the SIV is most evident due to the large number of of insulin receptors in the septum of the heart. Bi-ventricular hypertrophy, rarely right ventricular, may be associated (44,55). Cardiac function may be impaired, particularly during diastole, due to reduced left ventricular compliance and altered left atrial dynamics secondary to myocardial hypertrophy (50). HCM can range from asymmetric septal hypertrophy in the mildest cases (Figure 38), to dilated HCM or even massive hypertrophy (Figure 39) and heart failure in extreme cases (62).Some authors recommend that every

NNMD should, if possible, have a cardiac ultrasound within the first 12 to 48 hours of life to assess cardiac function and detect the presence of structural malformations (21).

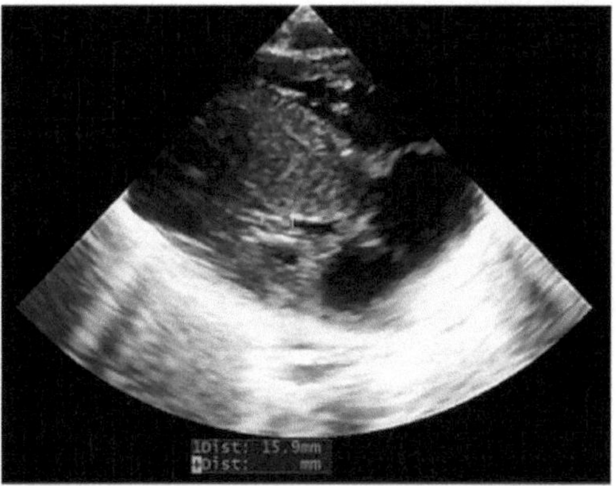

Figure 2: Postnatal echocardiography showing severe left ventricular hypertrophy and septal hypertrophy at 15.9 mm (78).

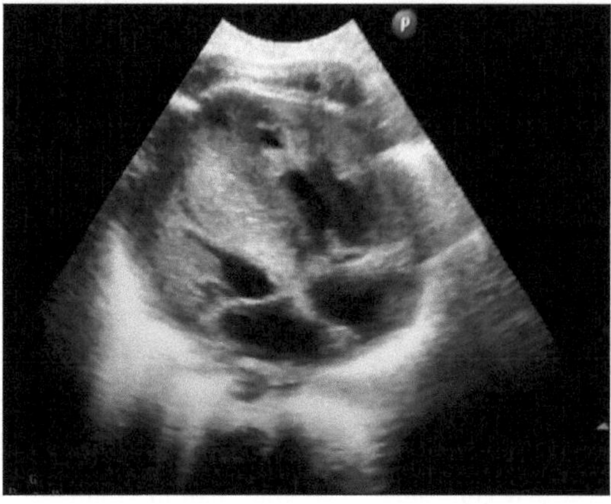

Figure 3: Post-natal cardiac ultrasound showing hypertrophy bi-ventricular with marked interventricular septal hypertrophy (30)

6.3.1. Ultrasound measurements

The various ultrasound measurements taken in our study were as follows:

- Left ventricular end-diastolic diameter
- Telesystolic diameter of the left ventricle
- Telediastolic thickness of the SIV
- Telediastolic thickness of the PPVG
- Shortening fraction
- Ejection fraction
- Obstructive nature

➢ **Telediastolic thicknesses of the SIV and PPVG**

The main parameter on which our ultrasound study focused was the telediastolic thickness of the SIV. The mean was estimated at 7.84 mm, with a maximum of 17 mm. The telediastolic thickness of the PPVG was the second most important parameter. in our study, with a mean of 5.19 mm. Demiroren et al (79) compared echocardiographic measurements between 83 neonates divided into 3 groups

- Group A: 33 NNMD
- Group B: 25 macrosomic neonates from non-diabetic mothers
- Group C: 25 eutrophic newborns

The ratio of left ventricular end-systolic diameter to left ventricular end-diastolic diameter in group A was significantly smaller than in group C. The ratios of SIV thickness (5.79 mm ± 2.04) to LVP thickness in groups A and B (1.29 mm ± 0.31 and 1.15 mm ± 0.19) were greater than those in group C. Vela-Huerta et al (80) studied the ultrasound parameters in 43 macrosomic newborns (22 NNMD and 21 newborns from non-diabetic mothers) and 70 eutrophic newborns. The mean thickness of the SIV in the 22 NNMD was estimated at 6.9 mm ± 2.8.

Septal hypertrophy was confirmed in 59% of them.

In another cohort collated by Vela-Huerta et al (1), the mean of

SIV thickness was estimated at 6.75 mm ± 1.75.

In the study conducted by Çimen et al (81), the thickness of the SIV in 16 NNMD was 8.75 mm ± 3.1.

➢ **Shortening and ejection fractions**

In the study by Vela-Huerta et al (80), ejection fraction (71.5% ± 7.8) and shortening fraction (36.6% ± 7.9) were lower in NNMD. On the other hand, in the series by Demiroren et al (79), the shortening fraction (41.8% ± 6.2) and ejection fraction (75.5% ± 6.8) in NNMD were higher than in controls. El-Ganzoury et al (23) studied cardiac ultrasound data in 69 NNMD. HCM was detected in 30 newborns (43.5%). Of these, 21 had SIV hypertrophy (greater than 4 mm) and 9 had SIV hypertrophy (greater than 4 mm) and PPVG hypertrophy (greater than 3.7 mm). It is important to note that this study detected impaired left ventricular contractility (shortening fraction less than 36%) in 52 NNMD (75.4% of cases). In the study by Çimen et al (81), the early diastolic, end diastolic and systolic velocities of the left ventricle, IVS and right ventricle were found to be significantly lower in NNMD than in neonates of non-diabetic mothers.

6.3.2. Characteristics of hypertrophic cardiomyopathy

In our study, obstruction was found in 34% of neonates. In the series by Narchi et al (71), obstruction was noted in 12% of cases. Indeed, five to ten percent of NNMD with HCM may develop reduced cardiac output due to obstruction of the left ventricular ejection pathway and reduced ventricular volumes (62). The obstructive nature was more frequent in our series since only symptomatic cases of HCM in NNMD were collected. In a study by Al-Biltagi et al (82), NNMD showed evidence of structural changes in the myocardium, with SIV/PPVG thickness ratios significantly higher than in controls.

6.3.3. Other anomalies

The cardiac anomalies most frequently found in NNMD are HCM and CAP (17).Noirin et al (18) studied cardiovascular abnormalities in NNMD between 2008 and 2010. The most frequently found anomalies were CAP, PFO and HCM. The same findings were reported in the study by Abu-Sulaiman et al (24). Zablah et al (51) studied postnatal cardiac ultrasound data in 631 newborns, 75 of whom were NNMD. There was a trend towards a higher prevalence of CAP in the NNMD group.

In the study by Vela-Huerta et al (1), echocardiography demonstrated a PAB in 15 of 33 NNMD with HCM.

In another study, Vela-Huerta et al (80) showed that pulmonary arterial pressures were higher in NNMD (38.5 mmHg ± 6.3).

Demiroren et al (79) noted increased right ventricular end-diastolic dimensions following supra-systemic PAH, whereas left ventricular end-diastolic and systolic dimensions were within normal limits.

FACTORS ASSOCIATED WITH SEPTAL HYPERTROPHY

7. Factors associated with septal hypertrophy

7.1.Maternal weight

Obesity in early pregnancy and morbid maternal obesity with a body mass index greater than 35 kg/square metre (m^2) are risk factors for congenital heart defects and HCM. A likely explanation for this is undetected maternal type 2 diabetes or gestational diabetes (4,70,83).

Obesity is an inflammatory disease. This inflammation causes endothelial dysfunction, arterial hypertension and insulin resistance (84). The various inflammatory proteins produced alter foetal systolic and diastolic function and lead to septal hypertrophy (85). Nyrnes et al (86) compared cardiac function between 55 neonates of obese mothers and 20 neonates of normal weight mothers. Cardiac function (systolic and diastolic) was impaired in the newborns of obese mothers, with a thicker SIV at birth and 8 weeks after delivery compared with the newborns of normal-weight mothers.

7.2.Type of maternal diabetes

In the study by Ullmo et al (7), foetuses of mothers with type 1 diabetes had the highest risk of developing HCM, followed by type 2 diabetes and only a small percentage in the case of GDM.

HCM was found to be significantly more frequent in newborns of mothers with gestational diabetes than with gestational diabetes (7.4% versus 1%) in the cohort conducted by Tabib et al (87).

In contrast, in the study by Vela-Huerta et al (20), HCM was detected in 54% and 44.4% of newborns of mothers with GDM and type 2 diabetes respectively, with no significant difference between the two groups.

According to a study carried out in Portugal (21), newborns from pregnancies complicated by GDM and requiring insulin therapy during the third trimester were 20.6 times more likely to develop cardiovascular problems than newborns from non-diabetic mothers.

7.3. Balancing maternal diabetes

The effect of strict control of maternal diabetes in preventing HCM remains controversial. In some studies, the incidence of complications has been reduced by strict control of maternal glycaemia (7). Fetal cardiac function is impaired when maternal HbA1c is high. Good glycaemic control would reduce the severity of dysfunction (88,89). El-Ganzoury et al (23) found that higher maternal HbA1c values (greater than 7.9%) were associated with an enlarged SIV. All newborns with HCM in this study were born to mothers with suboptimally controlled diabetes (HbA1c greater than or equal to 7%). Gonzalez et al (90) have shown that HCM occurs in 22% of pregnancies complicated by GDM, with a higher incidence rate for an HbA1c level above 7% than for a level below 5.9% in the third trimester. Russel et al (3) compared fetal cardiac ultrasound data in two groups of mothers followed for a PPD: well-balanced diabetes (HbA1c less than 7%) and poorly-balanced diabetes (HbA1c greater than 7%). There was no difference between the 2 groups during the first or third trimester of pregnancy. However, during the second trimester, isovolumic relaxation time and myocardial perfusion index were increased in women with poorly controlled diabetes. This is consistent with poorer cardiac function in the poorly controlled cohort. Although septal hypertrophy is less common in newborns from mothers with well-controlled diabetes, other studies have shown that HCM can occur even with good glycaemic control (5,13,91,92). The mean HbA1c level was significantly higher in the mothers of fetuses with septal hypertrophy in the study by Fouda et al (55). However, nine fetuses with septal hypertrophy had mothers with normal HbA1c levels. Weiner et al (92) found that the thickness of the SIV was greater from 22ème weeks of amenorrhoea to term in the foetuses of women with GDM whose glycaemia was well regulated (HbA1c less than 6.5%) in a prospective longitudinal study. In the study by Aman et al (67), no association was found between maternal HbA1c at the beginning or end of pregnancy and SIV thickness. Al-Biltagi et al (82) found no significant difference in global ventricular function between neonates of poorly controlled and well controlled diabetic mothers. In the study conducted by Vela-Huerta et al (20), no difference was observed in the frequency of HCM between the newborns of mothers with HbA1c levels above 6% and those with levels below 6% (60.5% versus 39.5%). To prevent HCM, glycaemic control may even need to be more rigorous than current recommendations. However, it is possible that other metabolic factors apart from maternal hyperglycaemia may be involved in the development of cardiac dysfunction. In hypoglycaemia the polycythemia and hyperbilirubinemia are found in up to 80% of NNMD (3,82).

7.4. Trophicity of the newborn

Several studies have shown a trend towards an increase in the incidence of MHC in high birth weight infants (23,24,70). In study by El Ganzoury and al. (23), the of echocardiographic measurements showed a highly significant progressive increase in SIV thickness, PPVG and ventricular dimensions with increasing birth weight. Birth weights above 3675 g were found to be significantly associated with an increase in SIV end-diastolic thickness. Rossi Palmieri et al (19) assessed foetal trophicity by studying foetal abdominal circumference. Half of the fetuses with a normal abdominal perimeter had HCM. The majority of fetuses (64.7%) with an abdominal circumference greater than the 75ème percentile had HCM. No association with the development of foetal septal hypertrophy has been established (50). This is consistent with the results of our statistical analysis.

THERAPEUTIC MANAGEMENT

8. Therapeutic management

8.1. Ventilation supports

NNMD have an increased risk of PAH. This is aggravated by hypoglycaemia, asphyxia and respiratory distress syndrome (93). Oxygen is a powerful pulmonary vasodilator. The increase in arterial oxygen pressure that occurs after birth is important in reducing pulmonary vascular resistance. Conversely, alveolar hypoxaemia increases pulmonary vascular resistance and contributes to the development of PAH. Oxygen therapy is therefore routinely used in the management of pulmonary arterial hypertension (94). In the study by Vela-Huerta et al (1), three of 33 NNMD with HCM showed echocardiographic evidence of left ventricular outflow tract obstruction. Two of these three newborns suffered heart failure and required mechanical ventilation. Nolent et al (95) reported the observation of a newborn from a poorly monitored pregnancy complicated by GDM. The newborn weighed 5100 g at birth. He presented with immediate severe respiratory distress requiring mechanical ventilation and nitric oxide without improvement. Cardiac ultrasound showed severe HCM with a SIV of 13 mm and significant PAH. The neonate was placed on extracorporeal oxygenation for 6 days and propranolol in doses of up to 2 mg/kg/day. He was extubated on day 20ème .

8.2. Pharmacological treatment

Treatment of HCM in NNMD is based on adequate physiological fluid intake and the use of beta-blockers. These block sympathetic stimulation and reduce heart rate. They increase filling time, reduce obstruction to LV ejection and reduce the heart's oxygen consumption (95,96). Propranolol is the drug of choice. It can be administered orally at a dose of 0.25 mg/kg/6 hours. The dose can be increased as required up to a maximum of 3.5 mg/kg/6 hours. Intravenous administration is also possible, starting with an infusion of 0.01 mg/kg/6 hours over 10 minutes and rising to a maximum of 0.15 mg/kg/6 hours. The drug should be administered under careful monitoring of blood pressure and heart rate (10).Complete relief of symptoms is obtained with standard doses of propranolol in 30% of affected neonates (71).

Inotropic agents (dopamine and dobutamine) and digitalis are contraindicated. They reduce the size of the ventricular chambers and worsen left ventricular obstruction (10,30).

EVOLUTION

9. Evolution

NNMD HCM is transient and benign in most cases. Clinical signs disappear after 2 to 3 weeks (30). In the study by Ullmo et al (7), 12 of the 92 NNMD presented with HCM, i.e. 13% of the cohort. Two deaths were noted: one had not adapted well to extra-uterine life and the other was due to heart failure. Cardiac ultrasound revealed concentric obstructive HCM with a SIV of 11mm, PAH, CAP and tricuspid insufficiency.

9.1. Developments during hospitalisation

In the study by Hăşmăşanu et al (22), the length of hospital stay was longer in NNMD (7 days) than in controls (5 days).

9.1.1. Hypoglycaemia

Transient hypoglycaemia in the postnatal period is the rule in all newborns, but tends to be earlier, more frequent and more severe in NNMD. This is more marked in babies born to mothers with unstable blood glucose levels at the end of pregnancy or during labour (97). In fact, 15 to 20% of NNMD present with neonatal hypoglycaemia (98). In the study by Ullmo et al (7), 48 of 92 NNMD presented with hypoglycaemia.

9.1.2. Hypocalcaemia

At birth, NNMD have a low increase in parathyroid hormone, resulting in temporary hypoparathyroidism. This hypoparathyroidism is linked to maternal and foetal hypomagnesaemia (62). It is generally asymptomatic but may be associated with agitation, lethargy, apnoea, tachypnoea or convulsions (10).

9.1.3. Jaundice

Hyperbilirubinemia is found in 20-30% of NNMD. Polycythemia produces immature red blood cell precursors which degrade more rapidly. This is exacerbated by hepatic immaturity and obstetric trauma (62).

9.2. Ultrasound evolution

All NNMD with septal hypertrophy should be followed by a paediatric cardiologist (62). Ultrasound normalisation is achieved after 6 to 12 months (30). Spontaneous regression of hypertrophy generally occurs when plasma insulin concentrations normalise during the first few months of life (99). MHC completely resolved in all newborns with MHC in the study conducted by Ullmo et al (7).However, the long-term consequences of neonatal HCM remain uncertain. There is little evidence on the impact of maternal diabetes on cardiac function in the offspring (100). Rijpert et al (101) studied cardiac dimensions and function in 30 children aged 7-8 years who were NNMD and compared them with a control group of 30 children of non-diabetic women. Echocardiography showed no difference in cardiac dimensions or function between the two groups. However, this study only included three children still being followed who suffered from neonatal HCM.

CONCLUSION

HCM in newborns may be the clinical expression o f various underlying disorders. The HCM of NNMD is a particular form frequently found in the offspring of diabetic women. Its pathogenesis remains poorly understood. However, it is postulated that foetal hyperinsulinism, secondary to maternal hyperglycaemia, may trigger myocardial cell hyperplasia and hypertrophy. These newborns were born to diabetic mothers. GDM was the most common (60%), followed by type 2 diabetes (22%) and then type 1 diabetes (18%). The average maternal age was 33.86 years, higher in women with type 2 diabetes.All pregnant diabetic women should be closely monitored during pregnancy, and in particular by foetal echocardiography.

Although generally benign and asymptomatic in the majority of cases, NNMD HCM may manifest clinically as respiratory distress, heart murmur, cyanosis or signs of heart failure.

Chest X-rays are the 1ère additional test of choice... Cardiac ultrasound is the most important additional test for confirming HCM and assessing its impact.

Therapeutically, the main compound used was propranolol. Hood oxygen therapy was the most commonly used modality. NNMD HCM is a transient disorder, with spontaneous regression during the first six months of life. This post-natal regression is linked to the normalisation of insulin levels. Regular cardiological monitoring with follow-up echocardiograms is necessary to assess the evolution of HCM. In short, despite efforts to maintain good blood sugar levels in diabetic mothers, HCM remains a frequent complication. Close monitoring of these pregnancies is essential. Much research should focus on foetal cardiac dysfunction and the ability to detect it early. Early detection of HCM in NNMD may prove invaluable for monitoring and delivery planning. The best way to mitigate the effects of diabetes on offspring is to prevent the development of diabetes itself. This can be achieved by preventing obesity before pregnancy, promoting physical activity and good nutritional attitudes. Optimising screening for GDM in pregnant women will enable early management and, subsequently, a reduction in perinatal complications. The role of good diabetes control in preventing HCM remains controversial. However, it may prevent severe forms. Future research should examine the necessary degree of glycaemic control during pregnancy to minimise the risk of HCM in NNMD.

REFERENCES

1. Vela-Huerta MM, Vargas-Origel A, Olvera-Lopez A. Asymmetrical septal hypertrophy in newborn infants of diabetic mothers. Am J Perinatol. 2000;17(2):89-94.

2. Elmekkawi SF, Mansour GM, Elsafty MSE, Hassanin AS, Laban M, Elsayed HM. Prediction of Fetal Hypertrophic Cardiomyopathy in Diabetic Pregnancies Compared with Postnatal Outcome. Clin Med Insights Women's Heal. 2015;8:CMWH.S32825.

3. Russell NE, Foley M, Kinsley BT, Firth RG, Coffey M, McAuliffe FM. Effect of pregestational diabetes mellitus on fetal cardiac function and structure. Am J Obstet Gynecol. 2008;199(3):312.e1-312.e7.

4. Chaudhari M, Brodlie M, Hasan A. Hypertrophic cardiomyopathy and transposition of great arteries associated with maternal diabetes and presumed gestational diabetes. Acta Paediatr Int J Paediatr. 2008;97(12):1755-7.

5. Ding F, Yu L, Wang M, Xu S, Xia Q, Fu G. O-GlcNAcylation involvement in high glucose-induced cardiac hypertrophy via ERK1/2 and cyclin D2. Amino Acids. 2013;45(2):339-49.

6. Reinking BE, Wedemeyer EW, Weiss RM, Segar JL, Scholz TD. Cardiomyopathy in offspring of diabetic rats is associated with activation of the MAPK and apoptotic pathways. Vol. 8, Cardiovascular Diabetology. 2009.

7. Ullmo S, Vial Y, Di Bernardo S, Roth-Kleiner M, Mivelaz Y, Sekarski N, et al. Pathologic ventricular hypertrophy in the offspring of diabetic mothers: A retrospective study. Eur Heart J. 2007;28(11):1319-25.

8. Malhotra A, Stewart A. Gestational diabetes and the neonate: challenges and solutions. Res Reports Neonatol. 2015;31.

9. Tests D, Diabetes FOR. 2. Classification and diagnosis of diabetes. Diabetes Care. 2015;38(January):S8–16.

10. Kallem VR, Pandita A, Pillai A. Infant of diabetic mother: what one needs to know? J Matern Neonatal Med. 2020;33(3):482-92.

11. Benhamida H. Cardiomyopathies in newborns of diabetic mothers: echocardiographic and Doppler analysis. Faculté de médencine de Monastir; 2009.

12. PICAUD J, CAVALIER A. Manuel pratique des soins aux nouveau-nés en maternité. Paris, France: Sauramps medical; 2008.

13. Maury P, Authenac C, Rollin A, Dulac Y, Mondoly P, Cardin C et al. Prevalence of early repolarisation pattern in children. Int J Cardiol. 2017;

14. Dubnov G, Fogelman R, Merlob P. Prolonged QT interval in an infant of a fluoxetine treated mother. Arch Dis Child. 2005;90(9):972-3.

15. Renolleau S, Rambaud J, Durandy A. Acute heart failure in children. Paediatric realities. 2014;27-30.

16. Pettersen MD, Du W, Skeens ME, Humes RA. Regression Equations for Calculation of Z Scores of Cardiac Structures in a Large Cohort of Healthy Infants, Children, and Adolescents: An Echocardiographic Study. J Am Soc Echocardiogr. 2008;21(8):922-34.

17. Paauw ND, Stegeman R, de Vroede MAMJ, Termote JUM, Freund MW, Breur JMPJ. Neonatal cardiac hypertrophy: the role of hyperinsulinism-a review of literature. Vol. 179, European Journal of Pediatrics. 2020. p. 39-50.

18. Russell NE, Holloway P, Quinn S, Foley M, Kelehan P, McAuliffe FM. Cardiomyopathy and cardiomegaly in stillborn infants of diabetic mothers. Pediatr Dev Pathol. 2008;11(1):10-4.

19. Palmieri CR, Simões MA, Silva JC, Santos AD Dos, Silva MRE, Ferreira B. Prevalence of Hypertrophic Cardiomyopathy in Fetuses of Mothers with Gestational Diabetes before Initiating Treatment. Rev Bras Ginecol Obstet. 2017;39(1):9-13.

20. Vela-Huerta MM, Amador-Licona N, Orozco Villagomez HV, Heredia Ruiz A, Guizar-Mendoza JM. Asymmetric Septal Hypertrophy in Appropriate for Gestational Age Infants Born to Diabetic Mothers. Indian Pediatr. 2019;56(4):314-6.

21. Bogo MA, Pabis JS, Bonchoski AB, Santos DC do., Pinto TJF, Simões MA, et al. Cardiomyopathy and cardiac function in fetuses and newborns of diabetic mothers. J Pediatr (Rio J). 2021;97(5):520-4.

22. Hăşmăşanu MG, Bolboacă SD, Matyas M, Zaharie GC. Clinical and echocardiographic findings in newborns of diabetic mothers. Acta Clin Croat. 2015;54(4):458-66.

23. El-Ganzoury MM, El-Masry SA, El-Farrash RA, Anwar M, Abd Ellatife RZ. Infants of diabetic mothers: Echocardiographic measurements and cord blood IGF-I and IGFBP-1. Pediatr Diabetes. 2012;13(2):189-96.

24. Abu-Sulaiman RM, Subaih B. Congenital Heart Disease in Infants of Diabetic Mothers: Echocardiographic Study. Pediatr Cardiol. 2004;25(2):137-40.

25. Jaeggi ET, Fouron JC, Proulx F. Fetal cardiac performance in uncomplicated and well-controlled maternal type I diabetes. Ultrasound Obstet Gynecol. 2001;17(4):311-5.

26. Australian Institute of Health and Welfare. Diabetes in pregnancy: its impact on Australian women and their babies. Diabetes series no. 14, Cat. no. CVD 52. 2010.

27. Helle E, Priest JR. Maternal obesity and diabetes mellitus as risk factors for congenital heart disease in the offspring. J Am Heart Assoc. 2020;9(8):1-9.

28. Devlieger R, Benhalima K, Damm P, Van Assche A, Mathieu C, Mahmood T, et al. Maternal obesity in Europe: Where do we stand and how to move forward: A scientific paper commissioned by the European Board and College of Obstetrics and Gynaecology (EBCOG). Eur J Obstet Gynecol Reprod Biol. 2016;201:203- 8.

29. Deputy NP, Dub B, Sharma AJ. Prevalence and Trends in Prepregnancy Normal Weight - 48 States, New York City, and District of Columbia, 2011-2015. MMWR Morb Mortal Wkly Rep. 2018;66(5152):1402-7.

30. Sharma D, Pandita A, Shastri S, Sharma P. Asymmetrical septal hypertrophy and hypertrophic cardiomyopathy in infant of diabetic mother: A reversible cardiomyopathy. Med J Dr DY Patil Univ. 2016;9(2):257-60.

31. Pauliks LB. The effect of pregestational diabetes on fetal heart function. Expert Rev Cardiovasc Ther. 2015;13(1):67-74.

32. World Health Organization. Global Report on Diabetes. Isbn. 2016;978:88.

33. Leirgul E, Brodwall K, Greve G, Vollset SE, Holmstrøm H, Tell GS, et al. Maternal Diabetes, Birth Weight, and Neonatal Risk of Congenital Heart Defects in Norway, 1994-2009. Obstet Gynecol. 2016;128(5):1116-25.

34. Walker A. Diabetes Mellitus and Pregnancy. J R Soc Med. 1928;21(3):377-85.

35. Lawrence JM, Contreras R, Chen W, Sacks DA. Trends in the prevalence of preexisting diabetes and gestational diabetes mellitus among a racially/ethnically diverse population of pregnant women, 1999-2005. Diabetes Care. 2008;31(5):899-904.

36. Cheung NW, Byth K. Population health significance of gestational diabetes. Diabetes Care. 2003;26(7):2005-9.

37. Ferrara A, Kahn HS, Quesenberry CP, Riley C, Hedderson MM. An increase in the incidence of gestational diabetes mellitus: Northern California, 1991-2000. Obstet Gynecol. 2004;103(3):526-33.

38. Mitanchez D. Neonatology: Scientific basis. Paris, France: Elsevier Masson; 2017.

39. Nguyen CL, Pham NM, Binns CW, Van Duong D, Lee AH. Prevalence of gestational diabetes mellitus in eastern and southeastern Asia: A systematic review and meta-analysis. J Diabetes Res. 2018;2018(Cc).

40. Nallaperumal S, Bhavadharini B, Mahalakshmi M, Maheswari K, Jalaja R, Moses A, et al. Comparison of the world health organization and the International association of diabetes and pregnancy study groups criteria in diagnosing gestational diabetes mellitus in South Indians. Indian J Endocrinol Metab. 2013;17(5):906.

41. Kessler J, Rasmussen S, Hanson M, Kiserud T. Longitudinal reference ranges for ductus venosus flow velocities and waveform indices. Ultrasound Obstet Gynecol. 2006;28(7):890-8.

42. Bilardo CM, Wolf H, Stigter RH, Ville Y, Baez E, Visser GHA, et al. Relationship between monitoring parameters and perinatal outcome in severe, early intrauterine growth restriction. Ultrasound Obstet Gynecol. 2004;23(2):119-25.

43. Zielinsky P, Marcantonio S, Nicoloso LH, Luchese S, Hatem D, Scheid M, et al. Ductus venosus flow and myocardial hypertrophy in fetuses of diabetic mothers. Arq Bras Cardiol. 2004;83(1):45-56.

44. Garg S, Sharma P, Sharma D, Behera V, Durairaj M, Dhall A. Use of fetal echocardiography for characterization of fetal cardiac structure in women with normal pregnancies and gestational diabetes mellitus. J Ultrasound Med. 2014;33(8):1365-9.

45. Davey BT, Seubert DE, Phoon CKL. Indications for fetal echocardiography high referral, low yield? Obstet Gynecol Surv. 2009;64(6):405-15.

46. Carvalho JS, Allan LD, Chaoui R, Copel JA, DeVore GR HK et al. ISUOG Practice Guidelines (updated): sonographic screening examination of the fetal heart. Ultrasound Obstet Gynecol. 2013;41(3):348-59.

47. Salomon LJ, Alfirevic Z, Berghella V, Bilardo C, Hernandez-Andrade E, Johnsen SL, et al. Practice guidelines for performance of the routine mid-trimester fetal ultrasound scan. Ultrasound Obstet Gynecol. 2011;37(1):116-26.

48. Asoglu MR, Gabbay-Benziv R, Turan OM, Turan S. Exposure of the developing heart to diabetic environment and early cardiac assessment: A review. Echocardiography. 2018;35(2):244–57.

49. Mongiovi M, Fesslova V, Fazio G, Barbaro G, Pipitone S. Diagnosis and Prognosis of Fetal Cardiomyopathies: A Review. Curr Pharm Des. 2012;16(26):2929-34.

50. Zielinsky P, Piccoli AL. Myocardial hypertrophy and dysfunction in maternal diabetes. Early Hum Dev. 2012;88(5):273-8.

51. Zablah JE, Gruber D, Stoffels G, Cabezas EG, Hayes DA. Subclinical Decrease in Myocardial Function in Asymptomatic Infants of Diabetic Mothers: A Tissue Doppler Study. Pediatr Cardiol. 2017;38(4):801-6.

52. Hatém MAB, Zielinsky P, Hatém DM, Nicoloso LH, Manica JL, Piccoli AL, et al. Assessment of diastolic ventricular function in fetuses of diabetic

mothers using tissue Doppler. Cardiol Young. 2008;18(3):297-302.

53. Eidem BW, Edwards JM, Cetta F. Quantitative assessment of fetal ventricular function: Establishing normal values of the myocardial performance index in the fetus. Echocardiography. 2001;18(1):9–13.

54. Friedman D, Buyon J, Kim M, Glickstein JS. Fetal cardiac function assessed by Doppler myocardial performance index (Tei Index). Ultrasound Obstet Gynecol. 2003;21(1):33-6.

55. Fouda UM, Abou Elkassem MM, Hefny SM, Fouda RM, Hashem AT. Role of fetal echocardiography in the evaluation of structure and function of fetal heart in diabetic pregnancies. J Matern Neonatal Med. 2013;26(6):571-5.

56. Zielinsky P, Satler F, Luchese S, Nicoloso LH, Piccoli AL, Gus EI, et al. Study of global left atrial shortening in fetuses of diabetic mothers. Arq Bras Cardiol. 2004;83(6):470-5.

57. Michael Weindling A. Offspring of diabetic pregnancy: Short-term outcomes. Semin Fetal Neonatal Med. 2009;14(2):111-8.

58. Weindling AM. The confidential enquiry into maternal and child health (CEMACH). Arch Dis Child. 2003;88(12):1034-7.

59. Yang J, Cummings EA, O'Connell C, Jangaard K. Fetal and neonatal outcomes of diabetic pregnancies. Obstet Gynecol. 2006;108(3):644-50.

60. Persson M, Shah PS, Rusconi F, Reichman B, Modi N, Kusuda S, et al. Association of Maternal Diabetes With Neonatal Outcomes of Very Preterm and Very Low-Birth-Weight Infants An International Cohort Study. JAMA Pediatr. 2018;172(9):867-75.

61. Cordero L, Treuer SH, Landon MB, Gabbe SG. Management of infants of diabetic mothers. Arch Pediatr Adolesc Med. 1998;152(3):249-54.

62. Hay WW. Care of the infant of the diabetic mother. Curr Diab Rep. 2012;12(1):4-15.

63. Persson M, Norman M, Hanson U. Obstetric and perinatal outcomes in type 1 diabetic pregnancies: A large, population-based study. Diabetes Care. 2009;32(11):2005-9.

64. Persson M, Pasupathy D, Hanson U, Norman M. Birth size distribution in 3,705 infants born to mothers with type 1 diabetes: A population-based study. Diabetes Care. 2011;34(5):1145-9.

65. Persson M, Fadl H, Hanson U, Pasupathy D. Disproportionate body composition and neonatal outcome in offspring of mothers with and without gestational diabetes mellitus. Diabetes Care. 2013;36(11):3543-8.

66. Lindsay RS, Westgate JA, Beattie J, Pattison NS, Gamble G, Mildenhall LFJ, et al. Inverse changes in fetal insulin-like growth factor (IGF)-1 and IGF binding protein-1 in association with higher birth weight in maternal diabetes. Clin Endocrinol (Oxf). 2007;66(3):322-8.

67. Åman J, Hansson U, Östlund I, Wall K, Persson B. Increased fat mass and cardiac septal hypertrophy in newborn infants of mothers with well-controlled diabetes during pregnancy. Neonatology. 2011;100(2):147–54.

68. Bhattacharya S, Campbell DM, Liston WA, Bhattacharya S. Effect of Body Mass Index on pregnancy outcomes in nulliparous women delivering singleton babies. BMC Public Health. 2007;7:1-8.

69. Usha Kiran TS, Hemmadi S, Bethel J, Evans J. Outcome of pregnancy in a woman with an increased body mass index. BJOG An Int J Obstet Gynaecol. 2005;112(6):768-72.

70. Al-Biltagi M, El razaky O, El Amrousy D. Cardiac changes in infants of

diabetic mothers. World J Diabetes. 2021;12(8):1233-47.

71. Narchi, H, Kulaylat N. Heart disease in infants of diabetic mothers. Images Paediatr Cardiol. 2000;2(2):18-37.

72. Kozák-Bárány A, Jokinen E, Kero P, Tuominen J, Rönnemaa T, Välimäki I. Impaired left ventricular diastolic function in newborn infants of mothers with pregestational or gestational diabetes with good glycemic control. Early Hum Dev. 2004;77(1-2):13-22.

73. Bacharova L, Krivosikova Z, Wsolova L, Gajdos M. Alterations in the QRS complex in the offspring of patients with metabolic syndrome and diabetes mellitus: Early evidence of cardiovascular pathology. J Electrocardiol. 2012;45(3):244-51.

74. Stern S, Sclarowsky S. The ecg in diabetes mellitus. Circulation. 2009;120(16):1633-6.

75. Maron BJ, Leyhe MJ, Casey SA, Gohman TE, Lawler CM, Crow RS, et al. Assessment of QT dispersion as a prognostic marker for sudden death in a regional nonreferred hypertrophic cardiomyopathy cohort. Am J Cardiol. 2001;87(1):114-5.

76. Arslan D, Guvenc O, Cimen D, Ulu H, Oran B. Prolonged QT dispersion in the infants of diabetic mothers. Pediatr Cardiol. 2014;35(6):1052-6.

77. Jorgensen M, Mcpherson E, Zaleski C, Shivaram P, Cold C. Stillbirth: The heart of the matter. Am J Med Genet Part A. 2014;164(3):691-9.

78. Codazzi AC, Ippolito R, Novara C, Tondina E, Cerbo RM, Tzialla C. Hypertrophic cardiomyopathy in infant newborns of diabetic mother: a heterogeneous condition, the importance of anamnesis, physical examination and follow-up. Ital J Pediatr. 2021;47(1):1-6.

79. Demiroren K, Cam L, Oran B, Koç H, Başpinar O, Baysal T, et al. Echocardiographic measurements in infants of diabetic mothers and macrosomic infants of nondiabetic mothers. J Perinat Med. 2005;33(3):232-5.

80. Vela-Huerta M, Aguilera-López A, Alarcón-Santos S, Amador N, Aldana-Valenzuela C, Heredia A. Cardiopulmonary adaptation in large for gestational age infants of diabetic and nondiabetic mothers. Acta Paediatr Int J Paediatr. 2007;96(9):1303-7.

81. Çimen D, Karaaslan S. Evaluation of cardiac functions of infants of diabetic mothers using tissue Doppler echocardiography. Turk Pediatr Ars. 2014;49(1):25-9.

82. Al-Biltagi M, Tolba OARE, Rowisha MA, Mahfouz AES, Elewa MA. Speckle Tracking and Myocardial Tissue Imaging in Infant of Diabetic Mother with Gestational and Pregestational Diabetes. Pediatr Cardiol. 2015;36(2):445-53.

83. Ece I, Uner A, Balli S, Kibar AE, Oflaz MB, Kurdoglu M. The effects of pre-pregnancy obesity on fetal cardiac functions. Pediatr Cardiol. 2014;35(5):838-43.

84. Bayoumy S, Habib M, Abdelmageed R. Impact of maternal diabetes and obesity on fetal cardiac functions. Egypt Hear J. 2020;72(1):10-6.

85. Cade WT, Levy PT, Tinius RA, Patel MD, Choudhry S, Holland MR, et al. Markers of maternal and infant metabolism are associated with ventricular dysfunction in infants of obese women with type 2 diabetes. Pediatr Res. 2017;82(5):768-75.

86. Nyrnes SA, Garnæs KK, Salvesen Ø, Timilsina AS, Moholdt T, Ingul CB. Cardiac function in newborns of obese women and the effect of exercise during pregnancy. A randomized controlled trial. PLoS One. 2019;13(6):1-19.

87. Tabib A, Shirzad N, Sheikhbahaei S, Mohammadi S, Qorbani M, Haghpanah V, et al. Cardiac malformations in fetuses of gestational and pre gestational diabetic mothers. Iran J Pediatr. 2013;23(6):664-8.

88. Gardiner HM, Pasquini L, Wolfenden J, Kulinskaya E, Li W, Henein M. Increased periconceptual maternal glycated haemoglobin in diabetic mothers reduces fetal long axis cardiac function. Heart. 2006;92(8):1125-30.

89. Turan S, Turan OM, Miller J, Harman C, Reece EA, Baschat AA. Decreased fetal cardiac performance in the first trimester correlates with hyperglycemia in pregestational maternal diabetes. Ultrasound Obstet Gynecol. 2011;38(3):325-31.

90. Gonzalez AB, Young L, Doll JA, Morgan GM, Crawford SE, Plunkett BA. Elevated neonatal insulin-like growth factor i is associated with fetal hypertrophic cardiomyopathy in diabetic women. Am J Obstet Gynecol. 2014;211(3):290.e1-290.e7.

91. Garcia-Flores J, Jañez M, Gonzalez MC, Martinez N, Espada M, Gonzalez A. Fetal myocardial morphological and functional changes associated with well-controlled gestational diabetes. Eur J Obstet Gynecol Reprod Biol. 2011;154(1):24-6.

92. Weiner Z, Zloczower M, Lerner A, Zimmer E, Itskovitz-eldor J. Cardiac Compliance in Fetuses of Diabetic Women. Obstet Gynecol. 1999;7844(99):3-4.

93. Seok H, Oh JH. Hypertrophic cardiomyopathy in infants from the perspective of cardiomyocyte maturation. Korean Circ J. 2021;51(9):733-51.

94. Fuloria M, Aschner JL. Persistent pulmonary hypertension of the newborn. Semin Fetal Neonatal Med. 2017;22(4):220-6.

95. Nolent P, Renolleau S, Hallalel F, Chevalier J., Costil J. Extracorporeal

oxygenation in a newborn of a diabetic mother with severe hypertrophic cardiomyopathy. Arch Pediatrics. 2002;9(3):271-3.

96. Dasgupta S, Qasim A, Aly AM, Jain SK. Mother With Diabetes Mellitus and Infant With Hypertrophic Obstructive Cardiomyopathy: Milrinone Precluded Need for Extracorporeal Membrane Oxygenation. Vol. 10, Circulation. Cardiovascular imaging. 2017.

97. Persson B. Neonatal glucose metabolism in offspring of mothers with varying degrees of hyperglycemia during pregnancy. Semin Fetal Neonatal Med. 2009;14(2):106-10.

98. Pollex E, Moretti ME, Koren G, Feig DS. Safety of insulin glargine use in pregnancy: A systematic review and meta-analysis. Ann Pharmacother. 2011;45(1):9-16.

99. Dasgupta S, Qasim A, Aly AM, Jain SK. Mother With Diabetes Mellitus and Infant With Hypertrophic Obstructive Cardiomyopathy. Circ Cardiovasc Imaging. 2017;10(11):1-3.

100. Marco LJ, McCloskey K, Vuillermin PJ, Burgner D, Said J, Ponsonby AL. Cardiovascular disease risk in the offspring of diabetic women: The impact of the intrauterine environment. Exp Diabetes Res. 2012;2012.

101. Rijpert M, Breur JMPJ, Evers IM, De Valk HW, Heijnen CJ, Meijboom FJ, et al. Cardiac function in 7-8-year-old offspring of women with type 1 diabetes. Exp Diabetes Res. 2011;2011.

SUMMARY

Around 3-6% of newborns born to diabetic mothers (NNMD) have cardiovascular abnormalities. Hypertrophic cardiomyopathy (HCM) is the most common cardiac disorder, accounting for 40% of cardiovascular anomalies. Its incidence, often underestimated due to the frequency of asymptomatic forms, varies between 30 and 40%. The HCM of NNMD is mainly induced by foetal hyperinsulinism secondary to maternal hyperglycaemia. It is characterised by disproportionate hypertrophy of the heart: hypertrophy of the interventricular septum (IVS) due to its high insulin receptor content, and free ventricular walls. Clinically, HCM may be completely asymptomatic, as seen on cardiac ultrasound, or manifest as congestive heart failure due to obstruction of the left ventricular ejection pathway. Whatever its severity, cardiac hypertrophy is transient, with echocardiographic resolution around six months of age in all cases. Treatment of HCM involves maintaining adequate fluid intake to ensure adequate preload and β-adrenergic blockers to slow heart rate and maximise diastolic filling time. Rarely, in cases of severe haemodynamic instability due to left ventricular failure and low cardiac output, haemodynamic support may be warranted. Milrinone may be useful in cases of associated PAH. Extracorporeal venous-arterial membrane oxygenation remains the last resort in the event of impaired cardiac output despite adequate management.

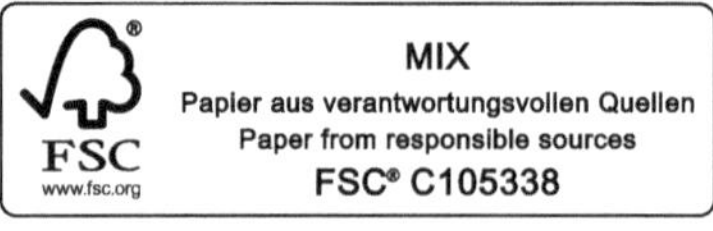

Printed by Books on Demand GmbH, Norderstedt / Germany